The Real Truth About Sugar

A Full Summary & Analysis of
Dr. Robert Lustig's Video Lecture
"Sugar: The Bitter Truth"

Samantha Quinn

TERMS OF USE AGREEMENT

The author and publisher of this book and the accompanying materials have used their best efforts in preparing them. The author and publisher make no representation or warranties with respect to the accuracy, applicability, fitness, or completeness of the contents of this book. The information contained in this book is strictly for educational purposes. Therefore, if you wish to apply ideas contained in this book, you are taking full responsibility for your actions. As always, the advice of a competent legal, tax, accounting, health or other professional should be sought.

ISBN-13: 978-1468161779
ISBN-10: 1468161776
First Printing, 2012

Printed in the United States of America

Copyright © 2011 by River City eBooks
4387 Swamp Rd., Suite 228
Doylestown, PA 18902
www.therealtruthaboutsugar.com

Thank You Gift

Thank You for purchasing this book. We appreciate your interest and have done our best to offer you an inspiring and practical guide to Dr. Lustig's video lecture and vitally important message.

Please accept a gift from us. Go to www.TheRealTruthAboutSugar.com/ThankYou to download some useful supplemental materials.

Thank you in advance for being part of our health advocacy efforts.

Samantha Quinn

& River City eBook

Foreword

Why a book that clarifies and summarizes Dr. Robert Lustig's viral video, "Sugar: The Bitter Truth"? That's easy. Dr. Lustig has quite likely identified the smoking gun for metabolic syndrome, type 2 diabetes, many forms of heart disease and quite possibly cancer. At the very least, he has identified one of the primary causes (or *the* cause, I'm sure he'd argue) of the obesity epidemic in America. This is perhaps the most important news in health care today, and despite the million plus views of his video lecture, Lustig's message isn't really being widely heard—or heeded. (To watch the video, click on the link given at the end of the book in References.)

The problem in large part is that his message gets somewhat lost in the medium. Ninety minutes long and full of charts and medical terminology, the lecture is held together for viewers largely by Lustig's charm and charisma. That much is perfect for video. The core message, however, may be very challenging for all but the biochemists in the crowd to really follow. Actually, that's not entirely true; we get what he is saying, that sugar is poison, but in all that detail we have trouble keeping the context clear and absorbing the enormity of his message. And how many of your friends, colleagues and family are actually going to watch the whole lecture?

A better medium for now spreading Lustig's message is the written word, and that is why I have written this book. We need to be able to see his ideas, findings and theories in black and white so that we can absorb it all. Re-reading a sentence or even a paragraph is no problem—we do it all the time to better understand things that can be challenging (and I have included time markers so that you may easily reference the video). This material deserves that kind of studious treatment. Lustig and other reputable scientists *know* that they are right about this, but until the long-term studies are done no one can claim that the evidence is conclusive. Lustig actually ventures out pretty far on his professional limb to give us this information, and we must do our part to take it from there.

Think about this: Did we really need to wait until all the studies linking smoking and adverse health effects were done to know that smoking harms us? Of course not. But the tobacco companies put us through the dog and pony show for decades and made it easier for us to deny or ignore the obvious truth and harder for our lawmakers to enact legislation. The truth is that we can expect the same treatment from those with vested interest in sugar and high fructose corn syrup sales. But we don't need to wait until then for us to start making wiser choices for our own and our loved ones' health when it comes to sugar. We can start today.

Alongside Dr. Lustig's work, I am including a chapter on Gary Taubes' New York Times Magazine article called "Is Sugar Toxic?" The reason for this is that Taubes gives us the larger context, in print, that Lustig is speaking from. In fact, I suggest that those who have not yet viewed the video start with the chapter on Taubes' article (or even read the original). This may even be a good approach for those who have viewed the lecture already. Taubes, an investigative journalist who has done extensive research in this field, offers the necessary background and punch for Lustig's claim that our sugar consumption is the source for much of what ails us.

Samantha Quinn, October 2011

Contents

Chapter 1

A Brief Overview

of Dr. Lustig's Lecture

Dr. Robert Lustig's "Sugar: The Bitter Truth" lecture video has been viewed on YouTube well over 1.7 million times. Why? Some would say that Dr. Lustig is an excellent presenter—charming, witty and fun to watch. This is all true. The real reason for the viral success of this video, however, is that Dr. Lustig has delivered compelling evidence for the difficult news that sugar is a poison. He claims that sugar is not acutely toxic, like arsenic, but chronically toxic, which means that its toxicity develops over a much longer period of time.

Two questions become immediately relevant: Is this really news? And: What's the bottom line?

The answer to the first question is no, and yes. In other words, we have long known that sugar is "bad" for us—even if we never really thought of it as a "poison." And there has been plenty of research to convince us that we should limit our consumption of sugar. The "yes, it is news" part of the answer is what need to pay attention to. Lustig (and others) are convinced that sugar consumption (specifically the fructose component of sugar) is the first step in the process of disease that includes metabolic syndrome, type 2 diabetes, obesity, many forms of heart disease, and possibly even cancer. In other words, our sugar (fructose) consumption is the culprit in what many see as the Western lifestyle diseases that have been meticulously documented throughout the world.

The second question (What's the bottom line?) is more complicated. We must first of all understand the cultural realities of the scientific community before we can grasp the scope of this issue. Lustig and others may be *convinced* that sugar/fructose is to blame, but they cannot say for certain that sugar consumption is the root cause of these diseases until long-term, double-blind studies have *proven* it to be so. Where does this leave us? The closest analogy to this state of affairs is to cigarette smoking. Until there were enough studies to overwhelmingly demonstrate the adverse effects of smoking, the tobacco companies were able to claim that there was no evidence that smoking *causes* anything harmful. They were able to point to contrary studies (funded by themselves) and to other possible causes (genetics, environmental issues, etc.) of disease to shield themselves from the legal and ethical consequences of their trade. To a degree, this continues today.

So what's the bottom line? The bottom line is that those with a vested interest in the sugar/fructose trade—from soft drink makers to breakfast cereal producers—will line up to fight any direct link between sugar consumption and health issues. This will of course slow down and water down the message that sugar is what is killing us in greater and greater numbers. Which means that the real bottom line is that we are going to have to decide for ourselves right now if the case against sugar/fructose is strong enough for us to make some perhaps radical changes in our food choices.

Concluding that sugar is a poison will have far-reaching, fundamental effects in our lives. As Gary Taubes in his New York Times Magazine article "Is Sugar Toxic?" puts it, knowing that sugar is not good for you is much different than understanding that "when you bake your children a birthday cake or give them lemonade on a hot summer day, you may be doing them more harm than good, despite all the love that goes with it." This kind of shift in our thinking will not come easily, nor should it be taken lightly. We have the responsibility to ourselves and our loved ones to face difficult truths, and to make choices for a better life even when it involves inconvenience and going against cultural norms.

That is where Dr. Lustig comes in. He is an MD, and is a University of California San Francisco Professor of Pediatrics in the Division of Endocrinology. Like a prosecuting attorney, he has presented his case, and we are the jury who is now weighing the evidence. So, let's take a look at his argument, given on May 26, 2009 for the UCSF Mini Medical School for the Public. As we already know, the title of the lecture is "Sugar: The Bitter Truth." What follows in this chapter is a brief summary of the lecture. Chapters Two and Three follow the lecture in much greater detail, and Chapter Four provides a larger context for Lustig's topic in part by examining Gary Taubes' New York Times Magazine article "Is Sugar Toxic?" (April 13, 2011).

―――

Lustig begins his lecture by stating his intention to debunk 30 years of nutrition information in the US. He then claims that the popular Atkins diet (all fat, no carbs) and the traditional Japanese diet (all carbs, no fat) both work for one reason: neither contains the sugar called fructose. Dr. Lustig refers to the National Health and

Nutrition Examination Survey (NHANES) Body Mass Index Data, which show that we are all 25 lbs. heavier than we were 25 years ago. He mentions that obesity is often seen as the consequence of genetic and environmental interactions, but points out that while our genetic pool has not altered much in the past 30 years, our environment has changed drastically. The conclusion he wants us to draw is that the rise in obesity is due to environmental factors, specifically increased sugar consumption.

There is a big mistake in how we think about food consumption, Lustig believes, and he likens it to a misinterpretation of the first law of thermodynamics in regard to human metabolism. Rather than our bodies either burning or storing the energy (calories) we consume, Lustig makes the point that there are biochemical processes that determine energy storage (weight gain). To counter this popular notion that obesity is a matter of diet and exercise, Dr. Lustig makes us aware that we actually have obese 6-month old babies—not just in the US but around the world. He claims that the common perception that if you don't burn the calories you eat you will store them (get fat) is patently incorrect, and he points to the obese infants as clear evidence for how wrong this popular idea is.

The problem, Lustig claims, stems from our negative feedback system being out of balance. Leptin, the hormone that comes from fat cells and informs the brain to stop eating, isn't working. Lustig says that we need to figure out why leptin isn't working if we want to understand the obesity epidemic. In the case of sweetened beverages, he suggests that the high sodium content is hidden by the sugar but still makes us thirsty.

So, what has changed in the past 25 years? While our genetics has remained unchanged in the past few decades, our environment has changed drastically, most especially the food we eat, how we eat, and how often we eat. Lustig reminds us that in the 1980s, the American Heart Association (AHA), the American Medical Association (AMA), and the U.S. Department of Agriculture (USDA) advised the public, in an effort to eliminate the occurrence of heart disease, to reduce the dietary consumption of fats from 40% to 30%. As we removed the fat from our diet, the incidence of obesity metabolic syndrome, non-alcoholic fatty liver disease, cardiovascular disease, and strokes actually increased. Lustig states that the culprit behind this is sugar, particularly fructose, of which we are eating more of today than we ever have before.

According to Lustig, when the fat was removed, sugar was added for flavor. He adds that sugar, commonly seen in products as either high fructose corn syrup (HFCS) or sucrose, can now be found in almost every kind of food-- from ketchup to pretzels. (It needs to be pointed out here that sugar—or sucrose—contains 50% fructose and 50% glucose, while HFCS contains 55% fructose and 45% glucose—making them, according to Lustig, metabolically equal.) Sugar is, however, most copious in beverages such as soda, fruit drinks, energy drinks, and even milk. Lustig refers to studies that have shown that excessive consumption of these beverages have been linked with obesity and Type 2 Diabetes. Another study conducted at the time of the lecture comparing schools with and without these high-sugar/fructose beverages show that schools without these beverages exhibit an unchanging prevalence for obesity, while in schools with these beverages the prevalence of obesity continued to rise over the year. Dr. Lustig shows that since 1977, consumption of HFCS or sucrose has doubled, comprising 12-15% of the total caloric intake for adolescents.

So why didn't a decrease in fat consumption lead to a decrease in weight? Sugar was added to make up for the lack of flavor in low-fat and no-fat foods, and we also greatly increased our portion sizes of sweetened beverages like soft drinks. The extra caloric intake, in other words, came from carbohydrates, not fats, and specifically the carbohydrate sugar. To make his point, Lustig calculates the weight gain possible from a daily soft drink habit:

Drink every day	Weight gain*
6.5 oz bottle of Coke	8 lbs. fat per year
12 oz bottle of Coke	16 lbs. fat per year
20 oz bottle of Coke	26 lbs. fat per year
44 oz. Big Gulp	57 lbs. fat per year

(*According to Dr. Lustig)

Lustig claims that sugar's prevalence in the market and our diet has been preceded by three major factors, which he terms "a perfect storm": the regulation of food prices in America, the invention of High Fructose Corn Syrup, and the advocacy of a low-fat diet. In 1972, with presidential elections at hand and in the midst of fluctuating food prices, Richard Nixon sought to de-politicize food as an issue and instructed his Secretary of Agriculture to find all ways to lower and stabilize food prices. In 1975, High Fructose

Corn Syrup was invented in Japan. Cheaper and sweeter than other sugars, High Fructose Corn Syrup caused the previously fluctuating price of sugar to stabilize in both the US and International markets. Finally, in 1982, the USDA, the AHA, the AMA told the public to reduce our fat consumption. This advisory came about after the discovery that the Low Density Lipoproteins (LDLs) found in our bodies increase with the consumption of dietary fat and correlate to cardiovascular disease. However, Lustig points out that this advisory was made without distinguishing between the two kinds of LDLs—Large Buoyant and Small Dense, one of which does not correlate with cardiovascular disease. The problem, Lustig explains, is that lipid profiles cannot distinguish between the two types of LDLs, so what matters is the triglyceride level. The ultimate result of this public advisory to reduce fat consumption is the low fat diet: high in sugar and fructose, low in fiber, low in trans-fats. Thus began what Lustig terms The Fructosification of America.

According to Lustig, to understand the true effects of fructose consumption, one must understand how it is metabolized. To do so, he compares fructose to both glucose and ethanol. In the body, only the liver can metabolize fructose—much like ethanol and unlike glucose, of which 80% is pre-distributed as energy to the other organs. As fructose metabolizes, it creates uric acid, which in excessive amounts can cause gout and hypertension. In the process, it becomes converted into xylulose-5-phosphate, which stimulates new fat making in the body. It ultimately gets packaged as Very Low-Density Lipoproteins (VLDLs), and because of the volume of calories, causes the dyslipidemia of obesity. Lustig states that a portion of the fat won't even make it out of the liver, causing a lipid droplet and in larger amounts, non-alcholic steatohepatitis. Another portion will come out of free fatty acids and will be retained in the muscle—telling the insulin to increase, raising blood pressure further, causing more fat-making, and affecting the way our brain reads leptin, hindering the hormone that tells your body that you've had enough food and can now burn energy. This creates a vicious cycle of hunger, more fructose, more carbohydrate, generating more insulin resistance. Ultimately, chronic fructose consumption creates hypertension, inflammation, hepatic insulin resistance, hyperinsulinemia, dyslipidemia, muscle insulin resistance, and obesity—effects similarly seen in chronic ethanol consumption.

Lustig points out that today, fructose is in everything we eat and drink, either as HFCS or sucrose. Soda contains about 10.5% per serving, and baby formula 53.2%. At McDonalds, Lustig claims that there are only 7 items on their menu that do not have it. Unfortunately, Lustig states, despite the effects of chronic fructose exposure on the human body, the USDA and the United States Food and Drug Administration (FDA) will not act on the problem. Because fructose is not an acute toxin but rather a chronic one, the FDA does not regulate it. He also calculates that the USDA cannot touch this matter because it would be an admission that one of the country's main exports, our food, is actually toxic. In the end, Lustig reminds us, the choice is up to us. Combating obesity and the metabolic syndrome start with the daily choices we make involving the food we eat and the lifestyle we live. For Lustig, this means greatly controlling our consumption of sucrose and HFCS.

Chapter 2

"Sugar: The BitterTruth"
—Part One

Obesity and High Fructose Corn Syrup

OBESITY: A GLOBAL ISSUE

Obesity is an epidemic we are all familiar with. We've heard the news, read the statistics and see it with our own eyes every day. According to Dr. Robert H. Lustig's data gathered from the National Health and Nutrition Examination Survey, we've greatly surpassed all previously predicted Body Mass Index levels by far. Obese or not, Lustig claims we all weigh 25 pounds more than we did 25 years ago.1 **(00:02:43)** Stated in his words, "the obese are getting 'obeser.'"

Lustig states that obesity is often considered the ultimate interaction between genetics and environment. Seeing as genetics has remained unchanged for about 30 years, according to Lustig, the escalating incidence of obesity can only be attributed to our vastly different environment. This, claims Lustig, is the point.

To understand obesity, Lustig suggests that we must first understand our view of it. For this he begins with the first law of thermodynamics, which holds that the total energy inside a closed system remains constant. When applied to humans, Lustig claims that we (erroneously) interpret it as the following: "If you eat it, you better burn it or you're going to store it." This common belief, Lustig points out, reduces obesity to two problems—calories in and calories out—and two behaviors: gluttony and sloth. Seen this way, obesity, as a condition, then becomes the fault of the obese person, a lack of diet and exercise. Yet if this is true, Lustig asks, then why are children in Tokyo, China, Korea, and Australia undergoing bariatric surgery? Why then are there obese 6-month-old babies? His point is twofold: no one chooses to be obese, and there are biochemical processes that determine energy storage (weight gain).

Therefore, according to Lustig, the First Law of Thermodynamics in regard to human metabolism should be stated: If you're going to store it, and you expect to burn it, then, you're going to have to eat it. Storing it refers to the biochemical processes behind energy storage, while burning it refers to the way our bodies expend energy and our quality of life. Lustig argues that in this formulation the biological processes are primary, ahead of any behaviors like gluttony and sloth. Seen this way, Lustig asserts that the obese person is actually more like a victim—which is how obese people actually feel.

Let's Talk Calories

According to Lustig, we are all eating more today than we did 20 years ago. He claims, using data from the US Department of Agriculture's survey[2] comparing the years 1989-1991 to 1994-1995, that teenage males are eating 275 calories more on a daily basis, adult males 187 calories more, and adult females 335 calories more. (**00:07:49**) This is where Lustig brings in leptin, which is a hormone that comes from fat cells. It tells the body when you have eaten enough and can now burn energy efficiently. If we're eating 187-335 calories more per day, then, Lustig claims, there must be something wrong with our body's biochemical feedback system. Our bodies should know when to stop consuming to maintain the right energy balance, which, Lustig implies, means that for some reason leptin isn't working.

So where are the extra calories coming from? According to data from the same source, only five grams or 45 calories out of 275 calories are from fat; the majority, 57 grams or 228 calories, actually are, according to Lustig, coming from carbohydrates.

In 1982, the American Heart Association, the American Medical Association, and the U.S. Department of Agriculture advised the public to reduce total fat consumption from 40% to 30%. And we did. Despite that, Lustig claims that obesity, metabolic syndrome, non-alcoholic fatty liver disease, cardiovascular disease, and stroke prevalence have all increased as fat consumption has gone down. In his words, "It ain't the fat, people." (**00:09:56**) It's all in the carbohydrates.

WHAT IS HIGH FRUCTOSE CORN SYRUP?
The Coca-Cola Conspiracy

Where do we get our carbohydrates? According to Lustig's data taken from the same USDA survey, we had a 41% increase in soft drinks and 35% increase in fruit drinks and fruit-ades just within that short span of time. With one can of soda equal to 150 calories, multiplied by 365 days a year, then divided by 3500 calories per pound[3], one can a day would directly translate to 15 pounds of fat per year.

Lustig traces the history of Coca-Cola to make his point. In 1915, the first bottle containing 6.5 ounces of Coca-Cola was produced out of Atlanta. Lustig claims that if we drank one of these every day a year, we would gain 8 pounds a year. In 1955, after the World War II, sugar wasn't being rationed and Coca-Cola introduced the 10-ounce bottle. According to Lustig, these were the first Coca-Cola bottles to be found in vending machines, and if we had one of these a day, this would mean an extra 13 pounds at the end of the year. In 1960 came the 12 ounce can, recognizable the world over. This was equivalent to 16 pounds of fat per year. In 1992, the plastic 20 ounce bottle was introduced, containing 2.5 8 ounce servings, worth 26 pounds of fat per year. Then there is the 7-11/Big K Thirst Buster Big Gulp product, a 44 ounce serving four times larger than Coca-Cola's original 10 ounce serving, worth 57 pounds of fat per year. Lustig reports that in Texas there is a Texas-sized Big Gulp—60 ounces of Coca-Cola, which is equivalent to 112 pounds of fat per year. (**00:12:25**)

Lustig states that Coca-Cola is composed of three main ingredients. There is caffeine, a mild stimulant and diuretic,

25

and salt, about 55 mg per can. The final component is sugar, which, Lustig believes is there in large quantity to mask the salt's presence and taste. When ingested together, this mix, Lustig observes, only makes you thirstier (a diuretic plus salt). In the 1980s, when New Coke was brought to market, the new formulation included even more salt and caffeine. This, claims Lustig, is evidence of the 'Coca-Cola Conspiracy' because "they knew what they were doing." **(00:13:32)**

The relation of soft drink consumption to obesity has been a controversial topic of study, with the results depending on who is performing the study. According to Richard Adamson, a scientist from the National Soft Drink Association,[4] "there is no association between sugar consumption and obesity." **(00:14:17)** According to Dr. David Ludwig, Lustig's counterpart at Boston's Children Hospital, data from their prospective study on softdrinks and obesity[5] have shown that "each additional sugar-sweetened drink increase over a 19-month follow-up period in kids increased their BMI by 0.24kg/m^2 and their odds risk ratio for obesity by 60%." **(00:14:21)**

Data from a meta-analysis, a rigorous statistical analysis of 88 cross-sectional and longitudinal studies regressing soft drink consumption against energy intake, body weight, milk and calcium intake, and adequate nutrition, all show significant associations. (**00:14:53**)

	Results	Reference
Energy Intake	0.16	P < 0.001
Body Weight	0.08	P < 0.001
Milk and Calcium Intake	-0.12	P < 0.001
Adequate Nutrition	-0.10	P < 0.001

On the other hand, when soft drinks were removed from the diet, the results were equally telling. Lustig states that during the Fizzy Drink Study[6] from Christchurch England, where soft drink machines were removed from the schools, preliminary data show that in schools where soft drinks were removed the prevalence of obesity remained constant, whereas in the control schools where the soft drinks remained, prevalence for obesity continued to rise over the year. (**00:15:24**)

Lustig also reports that another study from the Journal of the American Medical Association[7] in 2004 investigated the relative risk ratio for Type 2 Diabetes of all soft drinks, cola and fruit punch. Their results showed a trend of frequent and increased drink consumption elevating the risk for Type 2 Diabetes. (**00:15:54**)

What then is in soft drinks? In fruit-ades and punches? Lustig: high fructose corn syrup.

High Fructose Corn Syrup: America's Favorite Additive

High Fructose Corn Syrup (HFCS) is a sweetener composed of both glucose and fructose in varying ratios. It is present in almost every food type imaginable—from cookies to milk to pretzels. According to Lustig, HFCS is popular because of its sweetness, measuring at 120 on a sweetness index of 100, in comparison to glucose which measures at 74, sucrose at 92 and pure fructose at 173. (**00:17:24**) Given this, we should be able to use less syrup to maintain sugar levels in products. Unfortunately, Lustig reports, we actually use more.

Relative Sweetness of Various Carbohydrates	
Fructose	173
High Fructose Corn Syrup	120
Sucrose	100
Xylitol	100
Tagatose	92
Glucose	74
High DE Corn Syrup	70
Sorbitol	55
Mannitol	50
Trehalose	45
Regular Corn Syrup	40
Galactose	32
Maltose	32
Lactose	15

Lustig observes that there has been much dispute surrounding HFCS, especially since the substance has been greatly demonized in the public. To combat its worsening reputation, the Corn Refiners' Association released a statement declaring that "Obesity Research Shows High-

Fructose Corn Syrup Metabolizes and Impacts Satiety Similar to Sugar." To this, Lustig wholeheartedly agrees. Sucrose, commonly known as table sugar, is composed of equal parts glucose and fructose. With HFCS composed of 42-55% fructose, the difference in ratio is quite minimal. To Lustig, these two substances are basically the same thing; bad, dangerous and equally poisonous.

In February 2008, Gavin Newsom, mayor of San Francisco, floated a soda tax. Since then, Gov. Patterson of New York has followed in his footsteps and people have started to talk about it. The logic behind this strategy, claims Lustig, is: "Obesity is a problem; kids are drinking soda. Let's tax it." **(00:20:59)** The problem with this statement, says Lustig, is that the problem with soda consumption is not the empty calories but rather the fact that HFCS contains fructose, which is a poison. In response to this, a press release from the Center of Science for the Public Interest clearly states, "We, respectfully, urge the proposal be revised as soon as possible to reflect the scientific evidence that demonstrates no material differences in the health effects of high-fructose corn syrup and sugar… The real issue is that excessive consumption of any sugars may lead to health problems."

Our consumption of fructose and sugar has not always been this excessive. According to Lustig, prior to the advent of food processing, the majority of our fructose consumption came from fruits and vegetables. Daily, we would have ingested around 15 grams of fructose and 30 grams of sugar. Right before World War II, when food items were not yet rationed, consumption was slightly elevated to 16-24 grams daily. In 1977, Lustig observes that we begin to see a jump in consumption, up to 37 grams or 8% of our total caloric intakes, double our pre-war consumption pattern. This upward consumption pattern only continues from here. In 1994, daily fructose consumption is at 55 grams, 10.2% of our total caloric intake. In addition, daily sugar consumption at this point, Lustig claims, would be double this amount, at around 110 grams daily because fructose is only half of the sucrose molecule, the other half being glucose. Today, adolescents consume almost 75 grams daily, equivalent to 12% of our daily caloric intake. According to Lustig's data, 25% of adolescents today consume 15% of their calories from fructose alone. Year by year, not only are we eating more food and more sugar, but also we are doing so as we cut the fat from our diet. And, Lustig emphasizes, people continue to get sicker. (**00:22:17**)

When did this start? According to Lustig, it came about as a result of the perfect storm, an amalgamation of three political winds: the regulation of food prices in America, the invention of High Fructose Corn Syrup and the advocacy of a low-fat diet.

In 1972, food prices were fluctuating constantly, going up and down then up and down again. This is Lustig's first political wind. Afraid this would be an issue for him in the pending election, Richard Nixon told then Secretary of Agriculture, Earl Butz, to find a way to make the issue irrelevant. Lustig claims that the only way to do so would have been to not only stabilize food prices but also to keep them low. And this is exactly what Earl Butz set out to do—find any means possible to lower the price of food.

The second political wind came earlier. In 1966, Dr. Takasaki from Saga Medical School in Japan invented High Fructose Corn Syrup. According to Lustig, the substance then went on to be introduced into the market in 1975. Once again, prior to that point, food prices were fluctuating in the both the US and International markets and so were the prices of sugar, notes Lustig. When HFCS was introduced, sugar prices began to stabilize and since then have been quite constant.

The reason for this stabilization, claims Lustig, is because HFCS is much cheaper, about half the price of sugar. In his words: "high-fructose corn syrup is evil, but it's not evil because it's metabolically evil. It's evil because it's economically evil, because it's so cheap that it's found its way into everything." **(00:25:27)** Hamburger buns, ketchup, barbecue sauce, milk—almost every processed food today contains high fructose corn syrup, claims Lustig.

According to corn refiners, the presence of HFCS has been a matter of substitution, with the sugar being replaced in processed food gram per gram over time. Unfortunately, says Lustig, that isn't exactly what is happening. According to the US Department of Agriculture's Disappearance Data of Annual Per Capita Availability of Sugar and HFCS chart, although year by year the general trend is that the amount of sugar being removed from the food diet mirrors the amount of HFCS added, the total amount of Sugar and HFCS consumed continues to increase year by year. In 1972, the total amount of sugar consumption was at 73 pounds per year. In 2000, total consumption was approaching 95 pounds per year. (**00:27:05**)

Lustig claims that this is because the USDA's data fail to account for one thing: juice. Juice is, after all, sucrose. Lustig then cites a prospective study performed on inner-

33

city Harlem toddlers performed by Myles Faith[8]. (**00:27:38**) Lustig's chart shows a bar graph with juice servings on one axis and per-point change in BMI z-scores on another. Bars on the baseline reflect the increase or decrease of the BMI z-score in the individual child over a given period of time. Their data show that the number of juice servings per day can predict the change in their Body Mass Index score per month. Five servings a day can elevate a BMI z-score by 0.020 monthly. Where then do these Harlem toddlers get their juice? According to Lustig, from the WIC—Women, Infants and Children, an entitlement program established during the Nixon administration. What began as a program to prevent failure to thrive has now become the complete opposite.

With juice incorporated into the original USDA data of Sugar and HFCS consumption, the data show that we are actually consuming about 113 pounds per year as of 2000. According to the Journal of Clinical Investigation, Lustig states that today we are actually each consuming 141 pounds of sugar per year.

The final political wind in Lustig's perfect storm scenario occurred in 1982 when the USDA, the American Heart Association and the American Medical Association advised the public to reduce the consumption of fat in our diet. Lustig argues that this advisory was predicated by the discovery in the 70s that in our blood we had something called Low Density Lipoproteins (LDL) and that consuming dietary fat led to its increased presence in our blood. Later in the decade, we also learned that LDL correlated with cardiovascular disease.

According to Lustig, the thought process behind this advisory was: "If dietary fat led to increased LDLs and LDLs correlate with cardiovascular disease, then dietary fat should also correlate to cardiovascular disease. If we eliminate dietary fat then we eliminate cardiovascular disease." (**00:33:23**) Lustig claims that the logic behind this is incorrect. He states that the logic presented in this thought process is transitive whereas in reality, only the contrapositive is transitive. This means that in fact, no cardiovascular disease correlates to no dietary fat.

Lustig traces this logic back to Ancel Keys, a Minnesotan epidemiologist who sought to investigate the cause of cardiovascular disease. In doing so, he performed the first multivariate regression analysis without computers entitled *The Seven Countries Study*. His study looked at data from the US, Canada, Australia, England, Wales, Italy, and Japan, and appeared in Time Magazine in 1980. The object of this kind of analysis is to single out the contributing effects of each factor in the occurrence of a particular outcome. In Keys' case, this was cardiovascular disease.

According to Lustig, data from his study linked the percent calories of fat consumed with the coronary disease death rate of the seven countries. His data showed Japan and Italy were the two countries with the lowest scores and moving up, England and Wales, Australia, Canada and the US at the top with the worst numbers for both values. (**00:33:42**) The problem with this, Lustig insists, is that the top countries in the study are not just 'fatoholics' but also 'sugarholics.' On the other hand, Lustig points out, the Japanese diet, with their rice, and the Italian diet, with its pasta and gelato, featured a lot of glucose but very little fructose. In his words, "…the fat migrated with the sugar." Even Keys' goes on to acknowledge the intercorrelation of the two in his work[9]: "The fact that the incidence rate of coronary heart disease was significantly correlated with the average percentage of calories from sucrose in the diet is explained by the intercorrelation of sucrose with saturated fat… Partial correlation analysis shows that with saturated fat constant, there was no significant correlation between dietary sucrose and the incidence of coronary heart disease." (**00:35:19**)

Lustig informs us that in performing a multivariate linear regression analysis, it is imperative that each factor is isolated to gain an accurate representation of its contribution to the desired outcome. In this case where fat and sugar are intercorrelated, not only did Keys have to perform the analysis holding fat constant and showing the sucrose doesn't work, but Keys was also responsible for showing that fat still works when sucrose is held constant. Unfortunately, he did not, and since executed his study manually (he had no computers), we are unable to check his work.

At the time, Keys' work had a rival named *Sugar: Pure, White and Deadly* by John Yudkin, a British physiologist, nutritionist, and endocrinologist. Written in 1972, in this book, states Lustig, Yudkin has accurately predicted what has to come to pass, in terms of sugar and its effects on the human body. Unfortunately, we based 30 years of nutrition education and information and policy on the former instead of the latter.

In the fat versus carbohydrate debate (Keys v. Yudkin), there is also the issue of LDL, or Low Density Lipoproteins. Lustig states that there actually two very different types of LDL, and this turns out to be significant in the case against sugar. The first type of LDL is called Pattern A or large-buoyant LDL. Due to the fact that this type of LDL is light, floating and large, is does not find its way under the endothelial cells in the vasculature to induce the plaque formation process. The second type, named Pattern B or small-dense LDL is small and densely packed, easily getting underneath the endothelial cells and starting plaque formation. It is this type, argues Lustig, that can lead to cardiovascular disease.

When LDL levels are measured in the bloodstream, both are measured at once due to the difficulty in distinguishing one from the other. According to Lustig, to best determine which type is prevalent within your LDL reading, we must look at the blood's triglyceride (the major form of fat stored by the body) levels. Low triglyceride levels, coupled with high levels of HDL, good cholesterol, indicate the presence of Pattern A, large-buoyant LDLs. In contrast, states Lustig, high triglycerides with low levels of HDL indicate Pattern B, small-dense LDLs. This technique, claims Lustig, can predict cardiovascular disease more accurately than merely looking at LDLs alone.

Lustig maintains that dietary fat raises your large-buoyant LDLs while carbohydrates raise your small-dense LDLs. Lustig shows that in 1982, when we took on a low-fat diet, we also took on a high-carb diet. Ideally, when a low-fat diet is cooked at home, we can control the fat content. However, when it is processed, low-fat processed food becomes quite tasteless. Knowing this, Lustig states, food companies added taste in the form of sugar. Snackwells are a prime example of this, 2 grams of fat down, 13 grams of carbohydrate up (4 grams of which are sugar).

In other words, Lustig believes that we added fructose because we wanted our food to taste and look better. However, in the same way sugar browns our food, Lustig asserts that sugar works on our arteries as well, causing protein glycation and crosslinking, which contribute to atherosclerosis. We removed the transfats. Finally, we removed fiber because we wanted to make food last longer, cook faster and travel better. Today, Lustig states, we consume 12 grams of fiber today—compared to 100 to 300 grams of fiber a day fifty thousand years ago. Today, our food supply is, in Lustig's words, "adulterated, contaminated, poisoned, and tainted on purpose." In the next section, he goes into the biochemistry of sugar.

---

[1] Science 299:853, 2003

[2] Children 2-17 yrs, CSFII (USDA) 1989-91 vs. 1994-95,
http://www.usda.gov/cnpp/FENR%20V11N3/fenrv11n3p44.pdf

[3] If you eat/drink 3,500 calories more than you burn, you will gain one pound of fat.

[4] BMJ 326, March 2003

[5] Ludwig et al., Lancet 2001

[6] James et. al, BMJ 328:1237 2004

[7] Schulze et al, JAMA 292:927, 2004

[8] Faith MS et. al, Pediatrics 118:2066, 2006

[9] p 262, *The Seven Country Study*

Chapter 3

"Sugar: The Bitter Truth" —Part Two

Glucose is NOT Fructose

Lustig's lecture can be summarized in this sentence: Fructose, often delivered through the vessels sugar (sucrose) and High Fructose Corn Syrup, is actually a dangerous toxin. Though similarly sweet, the substance fructose is vastly different from glucose (the other half of the sucrose or HFCS molecule), Lustig explains, simply because of the way it affects our livers and bodies as we metabolize it.

Moreover, Lustig informs us that fructose is seven times more likely to cause a browning reaction in our arteries through a process called glycation, the very same process which causes to meat to brown on the grill.

Fructose also fails to suppress the hunger hormone, 'ghrelin,' as Lustig explains in detail. When ghrelin is not suppressed, we eat more. In the case of fructose consumption, this happens because there is no receptor or transport for fructose on the beta cell that stimulates insulin, and therefore insulin is not secreted. Because there is no insulin, explains Lustig, leptin, another hormone, does not increase. If leptin does not increase, ghrelin is not suppressed, and the brain doesn't see that we've eaten anything. Put simply, we eat more because we don't feel as if we've eaten anything.

The last and most important point Lustig makes in this regard is that liver hepatic fructose metabolism is vastly different from the way our bodies metabolize glucose. He claims that "chronic fructose exposure alone" is the cause of metabolic syndrome, a mix of the conditions obesity, type-2 diabetes, cardiovascular disease, lipid problems and hypertension currently affecting an estimated 75 million people in the United States alone. **(0:44:54)**

GLUCOSE/ETHANOL/FRUCTOSE:
A COMPARATIVE DEMONSTRATION

To truly understand the effects of fructose consumption on the body, it is necessary to compare it with similar substances and to take a close look at the biochemical effects each creates in the body. In this case, Lustig compares fructose consumption with glucose and ethanol consumption.

Glucose

For the purposes of this comparative demonstration, Lustig first shows us the effects of glucose consumption that come from ingesting 120 calories of Glucose—two slices of white bread.

According to Lustig, 80% of these calories will be used immediately by the other organs in the body. Every cell in the body, every bacteria and every living thing can use glucose. The remaining 20% or 24 calories will then be transported to the liver.

The Glucose arrives at the liver through the aptly named transporter GLUT2, or Glucose Transporter 2. Once in the liver, glucose stimulates the pancreas to make insulin. The insulin then binds to its receptor, IRS-1 (Insulin Receptor Substrate). A phosphate is added to this substrate via tyrosine phosphorylation, creating tyrosine IRS-1, which is active. This tyrosine IRS-1 then stimulates a second messenger called AKT, which in turn stimulates SREBP1 or Sterol Receptor Binding Protein Number 1.

Lustig explains that SREBP1 is ultimately the protein responsible for starting the fat making process. SREBP1 activates glucokinase, an enzyme that brings glucose to Glucose 6-phosphate. In this form, the glucose as Glucose 6-phosphate can only leave the liver through hormones, glucagon or epinephrine. However, as there are only 24 calories of the material, Lustig assures us that this is not a problem. **(0:46:48)**

To be stored properly, almost all Glucose 6-phosphate is converted to glycogen, its storage form in the liver. Unlike its previous form, glycogen can be easily removed using glucagon and epinephrine. According to Lustig, because glycogen is non-toxic, an unlimited amount can be stored within the liver. He confirms this with the example of children with "glycogen storage disease type 1-A" or "von Gierke's disease." Affected children with the disease (where Glucose cannot be removed from glycogen) may have swollen livers and be hypoglycemic, but they don't go into liver failure because "glycogen is a non-toxic storage form of glucose in the liver." **(0:47:37)** In fact, Lustig informs us, "The whole goal of glucose is to replete your glycogen."

During the conversion process, not all of the glucose is converted into *glycogen*. Some of the Glucose will be metabolized into "*pyruvates*." These pyruvates will in turn enter the mitochondria, the cells' energy-burning factories.

44

Within the mitochondria, the *pyruvate* is converted first into *acetyl CoA* during the Kreb's Cycle and the Tricarboxlyic Acid (TCA) Cycle and then is ultimately processed into *ATP* or *adenosine triphosphates* and carbon dioxide. We then exhale the carbon dioxide—which *is why* Lustig refers to *ATP* as the energy of life.

During the TCA cycle, when the majority of the *acetyl CoA* gets burned off, a minor amount of this substance may exit as *citrate*, leaving the mitochondria in a process Lustig calls the "citrate shuttle." According to Lustig, this *citrate* can then be broken down through three enzymes under *SREBP1*, namely: *ATP citrate lyase (ACL), acetyl-CoA carboxylase (ACC), fatty acid synthase (FAS)*. He further emphasizes that together these three enzymes are responsible for the de novo lipogenesis or new fat making process. Once broken down, Lustig states, we are left with *acyl-CoA,* which when packaged with MTP or Mitochondrial Trifunctional Protein creates VLDL or Very Low Density Lipoproteins. **(0:49:30)** VLDLs are known to form the base for adipose deposition in the fat cell and have been linked to heart disease and obesity. However, Lustig insists that at this stage, only around half a calorie of VLDL is produced from the original 24 calories processed by the liver. These levels, he says, are quite normal.

Earlier on, Lustig demonstrated when and how insulin secretion is triggered during glucose metabolism. The brain recognizes the raised insulin levels as a signal that the body has eaten and can now stop eating. This last stage is the most important, as it creates a feedback loop between glucose consumption, the liver, the pancreas, and the brain, keeping our bodies within healthy and normal energy balance.

In summation, the metabolic process of glucose consumption perfectly exhibits what is supposed to happen with our bodies. Energy from the food we eat is used by all the organs. What is extra is further processed in our livers for storage, either as glycogen or VLDL. During glucose processing, insulin is secreted, telling our bodies to stop eating. The body functions smoothly and at a normal, consistent level. This, according to Lustig, is good.

Ethanol

Next, Lustig discusses the metabolic processes of another carbohydrate, ethanol, commonly known as drinking alcohol.

Ethanol, like fructose and glucose, is a carbohydrate, composed of carbon, hydrogen, and oxygen. Ethanol,

Lustig reminds us, is also a toxin. Lustig details that acute Ethanol exposure can have the following effects: Central Nervous System Depression (CNS) depression, vasodilatation or the widening of blood vessels, hypothermia, tachycardia or increased heart rate during rest periods, myocardial depression, papillary responses, respiratory depression, diuresis, hypoglycemia, and loss of fine motor control. For those who drink, these are effects we have all felt firsthand at one point or another.

Conversely, acute Fructose consumption *has no immediate effect on the body*. Lustig explains that this is due to the fact that fructose, unlike alcohol or Ethanol, does not get metabolized in the brain, but rather, in the liver. Thus, we can conclude that fructose is not an acute toxin like ethanol.

Because we know that it is toxic, ethanol is strictly controlled. We have legal age limits, a Bureau of Alcohol, Tobacco, and Firearms, and taxes. According to Lustig, in Nordic countries, liquor stores are government-run in hopes of discouraging consumption through high prices. This is done for public health reasons. He points out that because we know that ethanol is a toxin, we have subsequently created over 1500 years of alcohol control policy in this world to limit its consumption.

To truly compare the effects of its metabolism, Lustig illustrates the metabolizing process of 120 calories of ethanol, equivalent to a shot.

Eighty percent of the 120 glucose calories (2 slices of bread) were used by the body before they hit the liver. With ethanol, ten percent of the ethanol will be initially absorbed by the stomach and the intestines while another 10% will be consumed by the kidney, muscle and brain, leaving 96 calories. In other words, Lustig shows us that the calorie ratio is now reversed. Instead of only 20% hitting the liver, here, only 20% of the original 120 calories has been removed. As a result, 96 out of the original 120 calories will enter the liver. This number is now four times the amount processed during the metabolism of glucose and therein, Lustig claims, is the problem. It's a matter of volume.

Because there is no receptor or transporter for ethanol, it enters the liver through passive diffusion. Once in, the ethanol is converted to *acetaldehyde.* Just like formaldehyde, *acetaldehyde* is bad for the body. Lustig explains that what *acetaldehyde* does is crosslink proteins, and too much of this activity within the liver causes cirrhosis, a condition where the liver cannot function because too much of its tissue has been replaced. *Acetaldehyde* also generates *reactive oxygen species (ROS),* which damages proteins in the liver. Lustig clarifies that the more alcohol we drink, the more ROS is created within the liver. The *acetaldehyde* will go down to a substance called *acetate*, which will then enter the mitochondria. **(0:54:29)** Similar to the pyruvate we saw earlier, the acetate will be converted to *acetyl-CoA* and go through the TCA cycle mentioned earlier to generate energy. Though alcohol may not contain nutrients, it does contain energy. As the *acetyl-CoA* is being processed, a much larger amount of *citrate* is being created and leaked off. Unlike with glucose, none of the calories is stored as glycogen during the metabolic process, so the full 96 calories also enter the mitochondria for processing. The much larger *citrate* created will be metabolized once again to *acyl-CoA* by the *SREBP1* to create a lot of *VLDL*. This, confirms Lustig, is the dyslipidemia of alcoholism.

In order to prevent itself from getting sick through fatty build-up, the liver will attempt to export all that *VLDL*. Lustig explains that some of it will exit as *free fatty acids* that then move into the muscles. Over time and with repeated occurrence, this will create Muscle Insulin Resistance, a condition where muscle tissue is slowly immunized from the effects of insulin, which then prevents the normal function of both your muscles and your liver and may potentially go on to cause other diseases, such as diabetes. Some of the *acyl-CoA* will actually be unable to make it out and will precipitate as a lipid droplet. Over time, the accumulation of these droplets can cause alcoholic steatohepatitis, a disease where the liver becomes inflamed due to fatty deposits.

Together, *acyl-CoA*, Ethanol and the reactive oxygen species from earlier activate an enzyme named *c-Jun N-terminal kinase 1* or *JNK1 (pronounced Junk-One)*. Lustig emphasizes that this enzyme is the main link between metabolism and inflammation in the liver and can go on to do serious damage to the liver.

In this discussion of ethanol metabolism within the body, Lustig clearly validates through his step-by-step explanation the fact that ethanol is a toxin, purely from the way it is metabolized in the body. He shows us that with ethanol the problems stem not only from the metabolic chain reaction it creates but also from the volume of calories to be processed. As the body is unable to use the majority of the ethanol it consumes, the liver is left as the sole organ capable of metabolizing it. The sheer amount of calories to be processed creates large lipid droplets and way too much VLDL, which subsequently creates fatty deposits and upsets how the liver functions. With increased consumption over time, ethanol could go on to cause serious liver disease, potentially escalating to complete liver failure.

As drastic as this is, Lustig then demonstrates that the metabolism of ethanol is not at all different from how fructose metabolizes and affects our body.

Fructose

As with ethanol and glucose, Lustig shows us fructose metabolism with 120 calories of sucrose, or a glass of orange juice.

First, Lustig reminds us that since sucrose is composed of equal parts glucose and fructose, there are about 60 calories of each substance in our glass of orange juice. Eighty percent of the Glucose or 48 calories of the orange juice are used by other organs, just as before. Of the original 60 calories, only 12 calories of Glucose are left for the liver. On the other hand, all 60 calories of fructose will be metabolized by the liver.

Lustig explains that unlike glucose and ethanol before it, only the liver can metabolize fructose. He goes on to state that foreign compounds that can only be metabolized by the liver, and which in turn generate multiple problems within the body, are classified as a poison. Using this definition, fructose, Lustig insists, can be labeled as a poison, and we can see this purely in the way it metabolizes, just as we saw with ethanol.

Because we know what happens to the 12 calories of Glucose, Lustig focuses on what happens to the 60 calories of Fructose as they arrive at the liver.

The fructose begins metabolizing by entering the liver through the transporter GLUT5. Unlike in Glucose, no insulin is stimulated upon entry. Once within, the fructose is metabolized by fructokinase to form Fructose 1-phosphate. In the process, phosphorylation (where a phosphate group is added to an organic molecule) occurs and ATP or adenosine triphosphate is relieved of one phosphate to create ADP or adenosine diphosphate. A scavenger enzyme called AMP deaminase takes the phosphates from the ATP molecule, converting them to ADP first then to AMP or adenosine monophosphate then to IMP or inositol monophosphate, finally creating uric acid as a waste product. Because, says Lustig, there are now 72 calories in the liver, instead of the 24 calories we saw earlier during glucose metabolism to be phosphorylated, the issue at hand is volume, just as in ethanol metabolism.

Conventional knowledge has it that uric acid is a waste product, excreted in our urine, commonly linked to the disease gout. Uric acid blocks "endothelial nitric oxide synthase," an enzyme present in our blood vessels that is responsible for generating "nitric oxide,' our internal blood pressure regulator, preventing our blood pressure from increasing. For this reason, Lustig believes that uric acid is also behind the disease of hypertension.

To illustrate the correlation between fructose, uric acid and gout, Lustig uses two charts (00:59:02) from a study currently in the NHANES database that was conducted by pediatric renal fellow Stephanie Win among adolescents.10 The first chart compares the amount of fructose ingested against changes in the serum uric acid while the second chart compares the amount of fructose intake with changes in the systolic blood pressure. Both these charts show that as sugar-sweetened beverage consumption increases, so does uric acid levels as well as systolic blood pressure. To illustrate the correlation between uric acid and hypertension, Lustig uses a chart (01:00:15) from a study conducted by Dan Feig at the University of Texas, San Antonio. Obese adolescents with hypertension were given allopurinol, a drug used to treat gout that decreases uric acid levels.11 Results show that during the course of this study, blood pressure, systolic and diastolic, decreased with the administration of the drug. This, states Lustig, shows just how big of a role uric acid plays in hypertension.

Regarding the current hypertension epidemic in the country, Lustig argues that "it's the sugar!"

Getting back to how fructose metabolizes, Lustig explains that fructose will be metabolized further into pyruvates, which, as we saw earlier during ethanol metabolism, will then enter the mitochondria and throw off a large amount of citrate. However, fructose does something unique when dihydroxyacetone-phosphate and glyceraldehyde reform to create Fructose 1,6-bisphosphate which will then reform once more with glyceraldehyde to finally form xylulose-5-phosphate.

Lustig interrupts the biochemistry lesson at this point to point out that sports drink companies use High Fructose Corn Syrup because it replenishes glycogen at a much faster rate than glucose alone. A faster glycogen replenishment rate is important because glycogen is burnt in the liver during intense physical activity, making High Fructose Corn Syrup a sensible component in sports drinks for elite athletes. Unfortunately, the issue, according to Lustig, is that elite athletes aren't the only people drinking these drinks. Children comprise a large segment of their actual consumers, and they do so because it's cool and the sports drinks taste good. Gatorade was first patented in 1967 by the University of Florida, and it skyrocketed in popularity, right after the Florida Gators won the NCAA football championship in 1970. The original patented Gatorade, the version sold at this time, Lustig notes, tasted horrible. Pepsi bought Gatorade in 1992, and in a quandary over how to market the product, added High Fructose Corn Syrup.

The thing here, Lustig argues, is that sucrose consumption leads to increased xylulose-5-phosphate. He explains that xylulose-5-phosphate stimulates PP2A, which then activates ChREBP or Carbohydrate Responsive Element Binding Protein, which in turn activates the three enzymes responsible for new fat making or de novo lipogenesis. (1:03:52) These three enzymes break down the citrate produced by the pyruvates earlier in the mitochondria. The process repeats much as before where acyl-CoA is generated and packaged into VLDL. Due to the volume of calories, Lustig states, we once again have the dyslipidemia of obesity from fructose consumption. A high-sugar diet, in other words, Lustig emphasizes, is a high-fat diet.

Lustig presents another chart in the video (01:04:27) of a study where normal medical students compared the impact of fructose and glucose consumption to de novo lipogenesis.12 The data is shown as a line graph with Fractional De Novo Lipogenesis and Time on the axes and glucose and fructose presented as lines on the graph showing changes over time. Ultimately, the chart shows that while very little of the glucose ends up as fat, around 30% of Fructose consumed does. Furthermore, when normal medical students were given a high-fructose diet over the span of six days, another set of charts (01:05:13) shows that not only was their de novo lipogenesis five times higher, but their triglycerides and free fatty acids doubled as well. 13 These free fatty acids, as Lustig states previously, go on to cause insulin resistance. Another study Lustig uses in the video (01:05:06) was conducted in 2005 and shows a link between the consumption of fructose and the increase in triglycerides.14 These data, argues Lustig, clearly show that when fructose is consumed, a person ultimately consumes fat and not carbohydrates. With this evidence Lustig makes his case that a high-sugar diet is in fact a high fat diet.

Returning to the metabolic process of fructose again, Lustig details how some of the acyl-CoA generated will create a lipid droplet, like with ethanol, once again potentially causing steatohepatitis over time, in this instance the non-alcoholic variety. Another study conducted within Lustig's clinic observed the relationship between sugar-sweetened beverage consumption and ALT or alanine aminotransferase, the liver enzyme marker which signifies a fatty liver. Their results show a definite direct correlation between the increase of sugar-sweetened beverage consumption and the presence of ALT, especially in Caucasians.

As we saw again earlier, Lustig explains how some of the VLDL will exit the liver as free fatty acids and populate the muscle, stimulating insulin while also creating insulin resistance in the muscle.

Lustig explains that acyl-CoA and the fructose activate JNK1. In glucose metabolism, IRS or Insulin Receptor Substrate becomes tyrosine IRS-1, which stimulates the secretion of insulin. With fructose JNK1 stimulates serine to phosphorylate with IRS1. However, the resulting compound serine IRS1 is inactive, which stops insulin's ability to perform its function in the liver. With insulin resistance in the liver itself, the pancreas works harder in order to generate higher insulin levels. A chain reaction within the body is set off where blood pressure increases, instigating raised fat making activity, and causes more energy to enter the fat cell. Thus, Lustig claims, the beginnings of obesity.

Furthermore, according to Lustig's research, the higher insulin levels are, the more difficulty the brain has in reading the hormone leptin. Our bodies continue eating because the brain fails to see that it has eaten enough or anything at all despite our fat cells generating stop signals. This change in the way our brains read energy creates an imbalanced state in the body.

At the beginning of the lecture, Lustig shows us a new way of viewing the first law of thermodynamics as applied to humans: "If you're going to store it and you expect to burn it, then, you're going to have to eat it." At this point, Lustig talks about the storage. (1:07:57) During normal metabolism, leptin should have been released as this point, sending the signal to the brain to cease consumption. It fails to do so because of high insulin levels and because of the nature of high fat diets. The body therefore continues to consume more carbohydrates and fructose, creating more insulin resistance, generating more fat, causing an increased imbalanced state and creating a vicious cycle of consumption and disease.

In summation, Lustig asserts that continued chronic fructose consumption can cause the following diseases: hypertension, inflammation, hepatic insulin resistance, hyperinsulinemia, dyslipidemia, muscle insulin resistance, obesity, and continued consumption—diseases that compose the metabolic syndrome. Compared to the conditions associated with chronic ethanol consumption—namely, hematologic disorders, electrolyte abnormalities, hypertension, cardiac dilatation, cardiomyopathy, dyslipidemia, pancreatitis, malnutrition, obesity, hepatic dysfunction or alcoholic steatohepatitis, fetal alcohol syndrome, and addiction—chronic fructose consumption also causes eight of those mentioned. This, Lustig asserts, is because they are the same and in fact come from the same place: ethanol is created by fermenting sugar. Despite the change is substrate, the basic properties have remained and can be seen in the metabolism of both.

Ethanol and Fructose are the same, Lustig argues. Both are poison. Both are toxins. (1:09:30)

AN INTERVENTION PROGRAM

Now that we understand the true nature of Fructose, Lustig asks: what can we do about it?

Lustig explains that in working with the rehabilitation of obese children, in his clinic they follow four main rules: eliminate all sugary drinks, eat fiber with carbohydrates, wait before second portions and exercise. These rules, states Lustig are very simple yet not always easy to follow.

As we learned earlier, sugar-sweetened drinks like soda, juice and sports drinks all contain considerable amounts of high fructose corn syrup and/or sucrose. These, in turn, create the considerable damage Lustig details in the second third of his video, not to mention the cycle of continuous consumption it creates. In order to rehabilitate successfully, children at Lustig's clinic are only allowed water and milk. As he says, "There is no such thing as a good sugared beverage, period!" (**1:09:50**)

The second rule is to eat fiber with the carbohydrates. Fiber is an essential nutrient that we removed from our diet to make food last longer so we can sell it abroad. Lustig says, "When God made the poison, He packaged it with the antidote." We clearly see now that fructose is a poison. In nature, however, wherever fructose is found, so is fiber—in greater quantities. He uses sugar cane as an example, a stick so tough the sugar cannot be chewed and must be sucked in order to be tasted. Studies on sugar plantations made during the early 1900s showed that plantation workers were actually healthier and living longer than the sugar executives and plantation owners who had access to the processed end products. In this way, fruits are okay. They limit the amount of Fructose taken in, have a degree of fiber and they provide essential micronutrients which allow the liver and the body to work healthily.

Lustig explains that fiber is important for three reasons. First, it slows the rate of absorption of carbohydrates in the intestine. A slower rate of absorption gives bacteria a chance to get to it first and break it down. This is not always good, according to Lustig—"it's either fat or fart." Next, fiber increases the speed of transportation of intestinal contents to the ileum, the final section of the small intestine. This raises the satiety signal hormone *PYY* and tells the brain that the meal is over. Fiber allows the food to move faster within the body, so we get the satiety "stop" signal much sooner, which chronic fructose consumption hinders. Finally, fiber inhibits the absorption of free fatty acids until the colon where these are divided into tiny fragments called "short-chain fatty acids." These actually suppress insulin instead of stimulating insulin, preventing issues with insulin resistance in the body.

Fiber is such a necessary element in the human diet and metabolic system that Lustig advocates a Paleolithic diet as the cure for type-2 diabetes. The Paleolithic diet involves eating everything raw—as it naturally comes out of the ground or from nature. Lustig states that the process would take about a week because we would be ingesting 100 to 300 grams of fiber. With fiber, Lustig says, "the more, the better."

Lustig's third rule in his clinic's intervention program requires waiting 20 minutes before getting a second portion. This gives the body time to process the food first and get that satiety signal out to the brain.

Finally, the last step in Lustig's intervention plan is exercise. In the case of these children suffering from obesity, he advises them to buy their screen or TV time minute per minute with physical activity. An hour of play equates to an hour of television time. This, he says, is usually the hardest step for these children.

Lustig refutes the notion that exercise is crucial because it burns calories. Twenty minutes of jogging, says Lustig, would only burn enough calories for a chocolate chip cookie. To attempt to burn off most of the calories we ingest would take so long it wouldn't be feasible on a daily basis. Consumption of a Big Mac would instantly equate to 10 hours of mountain biking!

Exercise is vital, first because it brings insulin levels down to healthy levels within the muscle by improving skeletal muscle insulin sensitivity. This helps in the prevention and combat against muscle insulin resistance. Lustig's second reason is that exercise is the body's natural stress reducer. When stress levels decrease, so does your appetite, as stress and obesity are intrinsically linked in a variety of ways. Finally, exercise can stop the creation of new fat by burning off the three enzymes responsible for de novo lipogenesis before they have a chance to become fat. Exercise makes the TCA cycle run at a faster pace so no citrate leaves the mitochondria to create fat and cause all the subsequent problems. This, explains Lustig, is what they call higher or faster metabolism.

These four rules give us an easy framework to take action, telling us what to do and why it is necessary. In practice at their clinical trials, Lustig finds that these four simple rules are very effective as treatment for their clinic's patients and results in a steady and positive change in the BMI scores. However, Lustig states that these rules would be ineffective if the patients continue to drink sugar-sweetened beverages. A multivariate linear regression analysis showed that the more the patients drank sugared beverages, the less effective the lifestyle intervention became. This result only further underscores the role fructose plays on the incidence of obesity and the metabolic syndrome.

---

[10] S Nguyen et al., Journal of Pediatrics

[11] Feig et al., JAMA 300-934, 2008

[12] Hellerstein et al., Ann Rev Nutr 16:523, 1996

[13] Faeh and Schwarz, Diabetes 54:1907, 2005

[14] Parks et al., J Nutr, 2005

Chapter 4

"Sugar: The Bitter Truth"—Part Three

Fructosification of America (& the World)

Now that we understand the impact of fructose on our bodies, the issue at hand then becomes: How do we avoid ingesting it?

Today, fructose can be found in almost every foodstuff, either as high fructose corn syrup or as sucrose.

According to Lustig, there are only seven items on the McDonald's menu without either of these two substances: French fries and hash browns are two of these items, containing only salt, starch from the potatoes and fat from the frying oil. Two more are sausages and Chicken McNuggets, although this only applies to the nuggets if they are eaten without the sauce. For the drinks, Lustig reports that there is no fructose in the coffee, Diet Coke and iced tea—but only if sugar isn't added. **(1:17:05)**

Fructose is most commonly found in the beverages we consume. Earlier in the lecture, Lustig reports that Gatorade contains a substantial amount of fructose. While this is actually beneficial for elite athletes, Lustig complains that they do not form the majority of Gatorade's actual drinkers. Gatorade's consumer group of children, for example, greatly contradicts its projected image. That is to say, sports drinks actually aid in the creation of more obesity than they do in the creation of world-class athletes. Lustig also questions the 112 pounds a year in orange juice given to schoolchildren in Salinas every day by the WIC—a government agency.

Lustig reports that some kinds of milk also contain fructose. Miriam, Lustig's young daughter, made a comparison of two cartons of milk: a 1% low-fat milk carton and a 1% chocolate milk carton, both from the same brand. The difference between the two was staggering. The 1% Low Fat Milk carton had 130 calories per serving, 15 grams of which were sugars, namely lactose. In comparison, the 1% Chocolate Milk carton contained 190 calories with 29 grams of sugar, the difference coming purely from High Fructose Corn Syrup. Lustig reports that what the San Francisco Unified School District has to say about this is: "Well, we have to get our kids to drink milk somehow."

Lustig contends that the epidemic of obese 6-month-old children that he referred to at the beginning of his lecture may have something to do with the amount of fructose found in baby formula. Currently, he reports, a can of formula is not only 10.3% sugar but also 43.2% corn syrup solids. Compared to 10.5% sucrose found in soda, specifically Coca-Cola, Lustig points out that there isn't much difference between the two substances. Furthermore, he claims that there is currently literature showing that the earlier children are exposed to sugar, the greater they crave for it later on. **(1:19:31)** Also, the greater the amount of sugar consumed by the mother during pregnancy, the more it permeates the placenta, altering the child's adiposity through "developmental programming" before its birth. In this way, we are actually creating the sugar craving and consumption cycle in our children from the womb.

Ultimately, Lustig emphasizes that there is no real difference between ethanol and fructose in terms of how the body metabolizes it. To show this he compares a can of Coke to a can of beer, both 150 calories each. A slide in his video provides the full breakdown. (**01:20:43**) In terms of carbohydrates, Coke is 10.5% sucrose, composed of 75 calories of fructose and 75 calories of sucrose. Beer, on the other hand, contains 3.6% carbohydrates of alcohol—composed of 60 calories of maltose and 90 calories of alcohol. First pass GI metabolism immediately skims off 10% of the alcohol, absorbed by other organs. Nothing is taken off for Coke. So, what now remains for the liver to metabolize, explains Lustig, are 90 calories from Coke and 92 calories from the beer. In other words, Lustig insists, there is practically no difference between the two—creating the same effect due to similar metabolism mechanisms with the same dosing. Yet, Lustig quips, parents would never give a child a can of beer. And, "Fructose is ethanol without the buzz." (**01:21:36**) Lustig argues that today, instead of "beer belly," America is suffering from "soda belly."

Lustig restates that fructose is a carbohydrate but that it is metabolized like fat. Studies he showed earlier on in the lecture tell us that almost 30% of ingested Fructose is metabolized into fat. In other words, repeats Lustig, a high-fructose diet is actually a high-fat diet. The problem, he argues, is that in America and around the world, what is known as a low-fat diet isn't really one because its sucrose and fructose content actually doubles as a fat. This is why our low-fat diets do not work—because in essence they are high-fat diets.

Knowing this, the inevitable question remains: what can be done about the problem? For those who are aware and have watched his lecture or read this guide, Lustig tells us how to live a healthier lifestyle in his intervention plan. What about those who have not, like the general public? What are the regulating food authorities doing? Not much.

Currently, FDA regulations state, according to Lustig, that "under the regulations governing food additives, it is required that additives be 'safe,' defined as a reasonable certainty by competent scientists that no harm will result from the intended use of the additive." (**01:23:23**) Lustig tell us that High Fructose Corn Syrup has GRAS or Generally Regarded As Safe status at the FDA. He explains that this comes from the notion that fructose is natural, found in fruits, and therefore it must be okay for consumption. He points out that tobacco and ethanol are natural, but they're not okay for consumption. Jamaican ackee fruit is also natural; however, ingesting it is fatal. Lustig reports that FDA regulations also state that "a food shall be deemed to be adulterated if it bears or contains any poisonous or deleterious substance which may render [it] injurious to health."(**01:24:15**) To this, Lustig argues, fructose definitely applies. However, notes Lustig, the regulation continues, "… but not with the prevention of chronic diseases even though its own regulations explicitly postulate the connection between such products and such diseases." (**01:24:26**) What this means, explains Lustig, is that the FDA allows high fructose corn syrup because it is a chronic toxin, not an acute toxin. Acute fructose ingestion does nothing except create fat. The liver gets sick after a thousand meals, not after one. Since fructose is in almost every commercially processed foodstuff available in the market, Lustig remarks, this "thousand-meal scenario" is actually a reality.

"What about the USDA?" Lustig asks. If the USDA were to impose strict regulations on our food regarding its fructose content, it would mean a public admission to the world that there is something very wrong with our food. Unfortunately, Lustig remarks, food is one of only four commodities America can still sell overseas, the others being weapons, tobacco and entertainment. The problem with this is that the USDA is currently in charge of the food pyramid, telling the public what is safe to eat. This, Lustig jokes, is the fox in charge of the henhouse! But unless the USDA changes its policy or its priorities, the public will continue to follow USDA advice until they are told or learn otherwise.

During the course of this lecture, our eyes have been opened to the true nature of fructose and its carriers, including sugar (sucrose) and high fructose corn syrup. As we've increased our fructose consumption, Lustig shows us that we have also created the obesity epidemic. Through him, we've learned that despite what experts try to tell us, a calorie is not a calorie. It's not just about how much we're consuming—it's really more important to see what we're consuming. What we consume makes all the difference. Lustig warns us that there are good fats and bad fats, good proteins and bad proteins. In the same way, there are good carbohydrates and bad carbohydrates; fructose is not glucose.

Through his lecture Lustig has also shown that Glucose is a good, healthy carbohydrat—the energy vessel of life. More importantly, we know now that fructose is a poison. Lustig has shown us that the metabolism of fructose leads to one or more of the conditions that comprise the metabolic syndrome: hypertension via uric acid, de novo lipogenesis, dyslipidemia, hepatic steatosis, inflammation through *JNK1;* hepatic insulin from the serine phosphorylation of *IRS1;* obesity and leptin resistance, promoting a continuous consumption cycle. In Lustig's words, "You are not what you eat" but rather, "You are what you do with what you eat." What our body does with fructose is dangerous and scary.

We know now that fructose is a chronic hepatotoxin, just like alcohol. However, because fructose does not get partially metabolized by the brain like alcohol, we do not get any of the instant effects acute alcohol consumption brings. In everything else, both substances are the same. But this lack of acute toxicity is exactly why the FDA and the USDA won't regulate it—in addition to the economic hit American producers would take if it were announced that fructose is a toxin that leads to metabolic syndrome and its host of disorders.

During the lecture, Lustig empowers his listeners to make better health decisions by way of sharing the intervention plan he and his team use at their clinic: exercise, eat fiber with carbohydrates, wait 20 minutes between portions and remove all sugar-sweetened drinks from our diet. He does so because in the end, it's up to us. The government is not going to save us on this one—at least not any time soon.

How we live and the choices we make, from how we eat to whether we decide to pay it forward, is what ultimately makes the difference, not only in our health but also in the battle against toxic food.

Chapter 5

Historical Overview
& Analysis

On June 2009, two months after the live University of California, San Francisco lecture, video of Dr. Robert Lustig's "Sugar: The Bitter Truth" lecture was uploaded onto You Tube. Since its first post, the video has received a total of over 1,700,000 views, gaining new views at a rate of over 50,000 a month. Gary Taubes in his April 2011 New York Times Magazine article "Is Sugar Toxic?" writes that these are impressive numbers considering that the video is a 90-minute lecture on the human metabolism of fructose. Taubes' article provides an interesting and useful frame for Lustig's lecture because it places Lustig's argument in historical context while explaining and developing its most important points. I will summarize the Taubes article here and suggest it as either a good starting point for those who have not yet watched the lecture or as an avenue for deeper study.

"Is Sugar Toxic?"

Taubes argues that the video's success does not stem from Robert Lustig's credentials as a specialist on pediatric hormone disorders and expert on childhood obesity, but rather from the nature and delivery of the subject matter itself. In the lecture, Lustig claims that sugar, in both its forms—sucrose and High Fructose Corn Syrup (HFCS)—is a "toxin," a "poison" and the primary cause of metabolic syndrome, a conglomerate of the highly prevalent diseases of Obesity, Type 2 Diabetes, Dyslipidemia, Cardiovascular disease and Hypertension. Lustig's insistence on this point, delivered publicly, expertly and compellingly, is what makes the video so popular and controversial, despite a number of critics who consider his case to be lacking in evidence. In "Is Sugar Toxic?" Taubes explores the different aspects of Lustig's argument and concludes that Lustig has the expertise and evidence to truly indict sugar.

Like Lustig, Taubes recognizes the importance of clarifying the term "sugar," as there has been much confusion about the two sugars sucrose and HFCS. Taubes explains that High Fructose Corn Syrup replaced sugar in the 1980s because at that time refined sugar had a bad reputation. He points out that during this period an article condemning sugar was published that was titled "A Villain in Disguise?" This bad reputation, coupled with the drastic price difference between the two sugars (HFCS being of course much cheaper), paved the way for High Fructose Corn Syrup's prevalence today. At present, the situation has been reversed. As High Fructose Corn Syrup is being demonized, sugar is once again replacing it in products. Despite the public marketing dispute, Taubes fully agrees with Lustig that both substances are identical in their biological effects and almost the same in their glucose/fructose composition, differing only in small percentages. In fact, Taubes tells us that High Fructose Corn Syrup was created to be "indistinguishable" from refined sugar. Taubes goes on to quote Luc Tappy, a researcher from the University of Lausanne in Switzerland considered by his peers to be the world's leading expert in the study of Fructose, that "there was "not the single hint" that High Fructose Corn Syrup was more deleterious than other sources of sugar."

How then, asks Taubes, does sugar affect our bodies?

In answering this question, Taubes draws from Lustig once more, stating that the concept of "empty calories" is the most common perspective regarding the consumption of food. In this line of thinking, sugar becomes a problem simply because we consume too much of it, not because there is something inherently wrong with how it reacts in our body. According to Taubes, this is the perspective taken by agencies such as the Department of Agriculture and the American Heart Association when they release advisories telling the public to cut back on sugar. Taubes then explains Lustig's main lecture point: fructose and glucose are "isocaloric, but they are not isometabolic"; they may contain the same caloric content, but fructose and glucose metabolize differently in the body--Glucose by all the organs in the body and Fructose wholly by the liver. Taubes maintains that while for some the jury may still be out regarding the effects of fructose consumption in humans, in laboratory mice it is accepted that "if fructose hits the liver in sufficient quantity and with sufficient speed, the liver will convert much of it to fat." If this effect is indeed the same for humans and we are consuming enough to create that effect, then our current lifestyle can only mean dangerous things for our health.

How Much Is Too Much?

According to Taubes, 2005 was the last year the government took an in-depth look at the implications and correlations between sugar and health. A report published by the Institute of Medicine of the National Academies recognized that a multitude of evidence was indeed present to support the claims that sugar elevates the possibility of heart disease, diabetes and even LDL cholesterol. However, the report also states that despite the plethora of research in this area, it is still not definitive; we cannot, with certainty, state at what levels sugar is acceptable in the diet and at what levels sugar becomes dangerous to our health. Taubes points out that these results mimic those of the Food and Drug Administration's report released in 1986, which said, "No conclusive evidence on sugars demonstrates hazard to the general public when sugars are consumed at the levels that are now current." While this statement neither refuted nor supported the case of sugar, Taubes notes that the Sugar Association and the Corn Refiner's Association took the findings to be an absolution of sugar at a time when sugar had a very negative reputation. To clarify things, Taubes refers to Walter Glinnsman, the primary author of the 1986 FDA report, who took the position that anything could be toxic if it were consumed in unnatural amounts. This question—how much sugar is too much?—is what Taubes examines next.

Unfortunately, Taubes notes, the 40 pounds per year used as the safe benchmark level for the FDA report is actually off by 35 pounds, at least according to the Department of Agriculture's estimates for that period. Taubes then makes reference to the compelling though circumstantial link between diabetes and sugar intake, pointing out that peaks in sugar consumption historically coincide with diabetes epidemics.

Going back to his earlier point, Taubes suggests that the way we treat sugar comes from our deeply entrenched belief that sugar is a sweet, safe additive. According to Taubes' research, this belief began in the 20th century when authorities were beginning to come to the conclusion that sugar was the cause of diabetes. Observing cultures where the use of refined sugar was uncommon, researchers noted the rarity of diabetes relative to its widespread occurrence in places and cultures using refined sugar, which suggested a direct correlation. Taubes also references Columbia University's Institute of Public Health director Haven Emerson's 1924 report that diabetes-related deaths had multiplied fifteen times in New York City and four times in other cities all over the country since the Civil War. Taubes notes that this spike in diabetes coincided with a significant upward trend in sugar consumption brought about by the birth of the candy and soft drink industries.

Countering Emerson's view was Elliot Joslin, the leading authority on diabetes during the time. Joslin's argument, explains Taubes, was that "the Japanese eat lots of rice, and Japanese diabetics are few and far in between; rice is mostly a carbohydrate, which suggests that sugar, also a carbohydrate, does not cause diabetes." His argument, though faulty, eventually won in the public debate. The problem, Taubes notes, is that two different kinds of carbohydrates do not metabolize the same way merely because they are both carbohydrates. Taubes emphasizes that Joslin could not know this at that time, just as he did not know that during this period the Japanese were eating very little sugar, in fact only as much as American consumption levels a century earlier. Unfortunately, Taubes reports, Joslin's constant repetition of his point of view eventually made his position on the matter the widely accepted truth.

After Emerson and Joslin, Taubes introduces Yudkin and Keys, two researchers Lustig also discusses in his lecture. Yudkin was the leading authority on nutrition in the United Kingdom, and, as Lustig mentions, published a book called Sugar: Sweet and Deadly. In this book, Yudkin presents the results from his feeding experiments on rodents, chickens, rabbits, pigs and college students. His research showed elevated triglycerides levels with sugar consumption, which subsequently elevates the risk for heart disease, and increased insulin secretion, which is linked to diabetes. Furthermore, Taubes explains that Yudkin also claimed that fat, whether saturated or saturated, was actually safe for consumption.

These are somewhat radical notions even today, and at that time Yudkin's views on fat directly contradicted consensus within the medical community that dietary fat was the primary cause of heart disease. According to both Taubes and Lustig, this consensus was largely influenced in 1970 by results published in Ancel Key's nutrition study The Seven Country Study. Taubes reports that Key's conclusion that saturated fat consumption is the best heart disease predictor was widely accepted. Yudkin's views, in this climate, did not fare well. Taubes quotes Jane E. Brody, a writer from The Times, who in 1977 wrote, "The theory that diets high in sugar are an important cause of atherosclerosis and heart disease does not have wide support among experts in the field who say that fats and cholesterol are the more likely culprits."

However, Taubes argues that much of the evidence for dietary fat as the primary cause for heart disease also make the case for Yudkin's sugar theory. During autopsies conducted on Americans killed in the Korean War, pathologists discovered that many had significant amounts of plaque in their arteries, whether they were young or old. Koreans, on the other hand, did not. The presence of these atherosclerotic plaques in Americans was immediately blamed upon their high fat diet while Koreans typically consumed low-fat diets. What they failed to see then, says Taubes, is that Americans also consumed high sugar diets while Koreans had low sugar diets. When Keys, a nutritionist from the University of Minnesota, published his "landmark" study in 1970, his results and hypothesis were accepted as compelling evidence for saturated fat consumption as a "dietary predictor" for cardiovascular disease. However, as we know from Lustig, the pattern of sugar consumption within the seven countries also mimicked the pattern of fat consumption, effectively becoming equally indicative of cardiovascular disease.

Lustig also indicts Keys for his meta-analysis study methodology since Keys failed to isolate the effects of his findings. While this doesn't make the case definitively for sugar, it does shed considerable doubt on Key's hypothesis, certainly opening the door for Yudkin's hypothesis. In Taubes' words: "It was possible that Yudkin was right, and Keys was wrong, or that they could both be right. The evidence has always been able to go either way."

To complicate things further, Taubes reports that there was animosity between the two camps. In 1971, Keys wrote a scathing article on Yudkin, his hypothesis, and its evidence, calling them "flimsy indeed." Scorned, Yudkin's public reputation never recovered, and all those who chose to study sugar and its effects were associated with Yudkin and treated in much the same way. Taubes quotes Sheldon Reiser, a scientist who attempted to do just that at the USDA's Carbohydrate Nutrition Library, "Yudkin was so discredited... He was ridiculed in a way. And anybody else who said something bad about sucrose, they'd say 'He's just like Yudkin.'"

Sugar and Metabolic Syndrome

Obviously, things have changed since then. Taubes writes that as Americans have gotten fatter and the incidence of diabetes has increased, "physicians and medical authorities have come to accept the idea that a condition known as the Metabolic Syndrome is a major, if not the major risk factor for heart disease and diabetes." Taubes points to data from the Center for Disease Control and Prevention that estimate that 75 million Americans now have metabolic syndrome. This is a staggering number.

Taubes explains the symptoms and pathology of metabolic syndrome. Typically evidenced by an "expanding waistline," metabolic syndrome has been associated with insulin resistance, where insulin isn't working as effectively as it should within the body. This means that as we eat, more insulin is required than usual to keep blood sugar normal after a meal. In time, as these elevated insulin levels continue to be secreted, the pancreas fails to "keep up" in terms of demand, or "pancreatic exhaustion" occurs. When blood sugar rises incredibly, we get diabetes. For those who do not get diabetes, other conditions may develop. Heart disease is one, where triglycerides and blood pressure levels increase and HDL cholesterol decreases, further fueling insulin resistance. In fact, according to Scott Grundy, a nutritionist interviewed by Taubes, metabolic syndrome is now the stronger predictor for heart disease than dietary fat ever was.

What then causes metabolic syndrome, or rather the insulin resistance that causes metabolic syndrome? Taubes explains that one of the prominent hypotheses among researchers in the field points to the accumulation of fat in the liver. Taubes quotes Varman Samuel, a researcher studying insulin resistance at The Yale School of Medicine, who observes that in the study of the link between liver fat and insulin resistance in humans, whether lean or obese, the correlation is "remarkably strong…. When you deposit fat in the liver, that's when you become insulin resistant." Although it is easy to suppose that a fatty liver stems from getting fatter, it is not that simple. According to Taubes, some cases of fatty liver can be traced back to "genetic predisposition," but there is a very strong possibility that Lustig is right, that it can be caused by sugar.

Apparently, the study of metabolic syndrome and insulin resistance are what lead many of the scientists currently studying fructose to become engrossed in the subject. According to Gerald Reaven, a Stanford University diabetologist whom Taubes references, fructose is one of the easiest ways to cause insulin resistance in rats, creating a "very obvious, very dramatic" effect. In the early 2000s researchers had "established findings" and "well-established biochemical explanations" for what was happening. Taubes phrases it as such: "Feed animals enough pure fructose or enough sugar, and their livers convert the fructose into fat – the saturated fatty acid, palmitate, to be precise, that supposedly gives us heart disease when we eat it, by raising LDL cholesterol." According to Michael Pagliasotti, a Colorado State University biochemist involved in many of the animal studies in the field, changes in the liver can happen within the span of a week if animals consume 60-70% fructose/sugar diets. If they consume the 20% levels of sugar/fructose found in American diets, the process expands to several months. As soon as the sugar is removed from the diets, the liver normalizes, and insulin resistance ceases to occur.

Taubes claims effects are similar in humans; however, studies in this area typically involve the use of pure fructose—as with Luc Tappy in Switzerland and Peter Havel and Kimber Stanhope at the University of California, Davis. The problem here is that pure fructose is not sugar or high fructose corn syrup. In Luc Tappy's experiments, Taubes reports, patients were fed the fructose equivalent of 8-10 cans of coke a day, "a pretty high dose" according to Tappy himself. At this dose, Taubes notes, their livers began to be insulin resistant and triglycerides would shoot up in a matter of days. At lower doses, the same results would appear but after a longer period of time.

Despite all the research, Taubes acknowledges that the evidence is far from definitive; the studies conducted on rodents do not really apply to humans. On the other hand, studies that were conducted on humans done by Tappy, Havel and Stanhope do not reflect actual human standards and experiences and thus do not apply; humans consume fructose with glucose, most commonly through sucrose or HFCS. Furthermore, our actual consumption of fructose is nowhere near the levels administered during these tests. Inconclusive results such as these are the reason why research reviews on the subject matter, such as those performed by the FDA, almost always claim that more research is essential, particularly research that attempts to determine at what dosage sucrose and high fructose corn syrup become "toxic." "There is clearly a need for intervention studies," Taubes quotes Tappy as saying, "in which the fructose intake of high-fructose customers is reduced to better delineate the possible pathogenic role of fructose. At present, short-term intervention studies, however, suggest that a high-fructose intake consisting of soft drinks, sweetened juices or bakery products can increase the risk of metabolic and cardiovascular diseases." Unfortunately, without long-term studies, definitive results are nowhere in sight. According to Taubes, it doesn't help that fructose is, as Lustig mentions, a "chronic toxin" and not an "acute toxin," "not toxic after one meal, but after 1000 meals."

Luckily, as Taubes mentions, there are several clinical trials currently running that are supported by the National Institutes of Health, all of which are small and short-term, lasting a little over several months. Lustig himself, together with Jean-Marc Schwarz, one of the best fructose scientists in the world, and their peers at UCSF are conducting one of these, studying the effects in obese teenagers of the consumption of fructose only from fruits and vegetables. Another study with the same consumption parameters will look for effects on pregnant women to see if healthier and leaner offspring are produced. To answer the main concern about levels where fructose becomes toxic, only one study is being conducted by Havel and Stanhope at the University of California, Davis, where healthy people are given three sugar/HFCS-sweetened beverages a day and to measure their impact on the body. However, the study's subjects are only observed for a maximum of two weeks, essentially covering only "42 of the 1000 meals," Taubes points out. Despite this, Taubes reports that the team is quite confident that the time period is enough to observe some symptoms of metabolic syndrome.

Sugar and Cancer?

Ultimately, Taubes concludes his inquiry on sugar on a familiar note: sugar could be toxic, it can have all the effects Lustig and Yudkin claim it does, but we do not know how much we have to ingest before this happens. Years could pass before sugar consumption does any damage, and until we study its effects in the long term, we may never know for sure.

Taubes, however, does not leave it at that, and he asks one last question: "What are the chances that sugar is actually worse than Lustig says it is?" He asks this because whenever the occurrence of obesity, diabetes and metabolic syndrome rises, so does the incidence of cancer. Taubes emphasizes that insulin resistance may also be an underlying factor in many cancers, just like in Type-2 Diabetes and heart disease. The links between the diseases was first noted by the World Health Organization's International Agency for Research on Cancer in their 2004 large population studies. However, Taubes reports that unlike the data against sugar, the link is not controversial, merely stating that cancer is more likely to happen if one already has metabolic syndrome. This fuels the commonly held view that many cancers are caused by Western diets and lifestyle. Taubes states that if this is indeed true, there may be a way to prevent its occurrence through isolating the trigger substance/condition.

This point of view is commonly accepted mainly because these are two main observations which support it. The first observation, Taubes explains, involves the jump in cancer death rates in end of the 19th to the beginning of the 20th century. Similar to the diabetes epidemic, this increase in the cancer death rate was heavily contested. In Taubes' words, the argument was about "whether those increases could be explained solely by the aging of the population and the use of new diagnostic techniques or whether it was really the incidence of cancer itself that was increasing." According to a 1997 report by the World

Cancer Research Fund International and the American Institute for Cancer, "by the 1930s…it was apparent that age-adjusted death rates from cancer were rising in the U.S.A"

The second observation is similar to Key's observations in the Seven Countries Study: In areas where Western diets were uncommon, so was the incidence of "malignant" cancer. Taubes claims that in the 1950s, cancer among the Inuit was so rare that should a case exhibit itself, physicians would immediately publish reports in medical journals for documentation. In 1984, cancer incidents among the Inuit were analyzed. Taubes shows that results of the study claimed a "striking increase in the incidence of cancers of modern societies" such as lung and cervical cancer, though in breast cancer rates there were "conspicuous deficits." Diabetes rates went from virtually non-existent in the '50s to high today.

Taubes notes that the majority of researchers agree that Western diet and lifestyle play a huge role in the incidence of cancer, and that it "manifests itself with obesity, diabetes, and metabolic syndrome." The root of the problem is the more insulin resistant we are and the greater levels of insulin we secrete, the more tumor growth is promoted within the body. Taubes references Craig Thompson, primary researcher in the field and president of Memorial Sloan–Kettering Cancer Center in New York, to explain: "the cells of many human cancers come to depend on insulin to provide the fuel (blood sugar) and material they need to grow and multiply. Insulin and insulin–like growth factors (and related growth factors) also provide the signal, in effect, to do it. The more insulin, the better they do. Some cancers develop mutations that serve the purpose of increasing the influence of insulin on the cell; others take advantage of the elevated insulin levels that are common to metabolic syndrome, obesity and type 2 diabetes. Some do both." Researchers say that this step is fundamental in many human cancers. In fact, 80 percent of these cancers stem from these mutations or from factors that either copy or enhance insulin's impact on the incipient tumor cells, says Lewis Cantley, director of the Cancer Center at Beth Israel Deaconess Medical Center at Harvard Medical School.

In finding a solution, Taubes reports that most researchers are focused on finding or creating an insulin-signaling suppressing drug that they hope can inhibit or prevent the growth of incipient cancer cells. Experts also suggest slimming down and working towards having more active lifestyles, since a common assumption within their community, especially World Cancer Research Fund and the American Institute for Cancer Research, is that insulin levels and resistance is caused by the fat or getting fatter. However, some researchers are willing to say, like Cantley and Thomson, that being fat and becoming fat may be just one aspect. If any food creates insulin resistance within the body, this may be the dietary cause of cancer. Taubes explains that if sugar does cause insulin resistance, then the next logical thought would be to connect sugar to cancer. He quotes Memorial Sloan-Kettering Cancer Center president Craig Thompson, who says, "I have eliminated refined sugar from my diet and eat as little as I possible can because I believe ultimately it's something I can do to decrease my risk of cancer."

As for Taubes, who has studied and reported on sugar for over a decade, he leaves us with this thought:

"Officially I'm not supposed to worry because the evidence isn't conclusive, but I do."

Thank you again for purchasing this book.

Please remember to go to:

www.TheRealTruthAboutSugar.com/ThankYou

to accept your free supplementary materials.

These materials may be copied and given away to personal friends and family members, but they may not be publicly distributed or sold.

Thank You! May you live well and be healthy.

References & Further Reading/Viewing

Sugar: The Bitter Truth. Robert H. Lustig, MD. Mini Medical School for the Public, 2009. University of California Television. Accessed 26 August 2011 <http://www.youtube.com/watch?v=dBnniua6-oM>

Keys, Ancel. *Seven Countries: a Multivariate Analysis of Death and Coronary Heart Disease.* London: Harvard UP, 1980. Print.

Marissa, Cevallos. "Sugar: The Toxicity Question and What to Do about It." *The Los Angeles Times.* 19 Apr. 2011.

"NHANES - National Health and Nutrition Examination Survey Homepage." *Centers for Disease Control and Prevention.* Web. Accessed19 Sept. 2011. <http://www.cdc.gov/nchs/nhanes.htm>

Taubes, Gary. "Is Sugar Toxic?" *The New York Times.* 13 Apr. 2011. Web. 22 July 2011. <http://www.nytimes.com/2011/04/17/magazine/mag-17Sugar-t.html?_r=2&pagewanted=print>.

Yudkin, John. *Sweet and Dangerous.* New York: Bantam Books, 1972

Yudkin, John. *Pure, White and Deadly.* Davis-Poynter Ltd, 1972.

Made in the USA
Lexington, KY
17 April 2016